Heart Surgery

And What They Don't Tell You

By Robert House

Contents

Introduction

The reason for this book is to tell **the rest of the story** about heart surgery, the after care and help you to know what to expect. It may seem to you that no one may take the time to tell you a lot of the things that will help to prepare you for what is to come.

In this first-person account, author Robert House examines his own recovery from open-heart surgery and the road back to health and fitness as an Open Heart Survivor.

In September 2014, Robert had chest discomfort and pain and ultimately had quintuple bypass surgery.

Looking back over the previous year, he recognized many times that he denied symptoms and ignored the possibility that his heart was in trouble. Following the surgery, Robert made a promise about his own recovery process so others could learn from it; and to get back in shape. From his point of personal view, it does require a great amount of determination and the mind set to persevere.

Roberts' story is for anyone diagnosed with heart disease whether they are treating their condition with their diet and medications, received stents to open arteries or are going to have, or already had open-heart surgery.

Yes, if you get to a certain stage you will be talking to a doctor about open heart surgery. It will be a scary situation knowing what may lay ahead for you. However, it is important to be positive, hope and expect for the best of results. This is still a very serious surgery and often a long recovery. There will be possibly many potential problems in the recovery process. But you need to be determined and press forward towards great health.

When faced with these symptoms often it is very stressful and difficult to make decisions. Granted it is a very scary time in any body's life and I hope and trust that you have loved ones with you during these times.

Typically all the nurses and doctors will be professional and dedicated to caring for your wellbeing. I can say that from my own personal experience, there were so many caring nurses and doctors that cared about my recovery and long term health.

I will attempt to give some important information that I experienced during my open heart surgery and recovery. There is some vital information that I was not aware of and can make a major difference in the outcome of our health. What we are after is the very best for our long term health.

I trust that you will find some words of wisdom and will benefit from this book. Remember that I am not a medical doctor or have ever had any training and **I am not giving medical advice.** This is my personal story of my experience with having an open heart by-pass and the recovery and the continuing after care. You should and must always consult a qualified doctor in any decisions that you make.

Be always willing to speak up, and ask questions about anything that you do not understand and when you think of something and the doctor is not there, ask someone to write in down for you so you can be sure to get your questions answered. Remember that the doctors and nurses have a lot of important things that they are dealing with.

Make a list of questions and make sure that these questions are answered and you understand the answer. Ask more questions if need be.

So what are my risks in this procedure and or surgery? Typically what is the outcome for my situation? Will I have a long recovery or will it be short? Will my lifestyle change dramatically? Will I still be able to play tennis? Will I still be able to have sex? Write your questions down.

I believe it is a great help to meditate or do whatever you find helps you to remain calm during these difficult times. I found myself to not be taking good breaths during the more stressful times and that is something to remain aware of, as it can make a difference in your stress levels. Stress is not your friend during this time.

If you are a religious person I recommend that you find someone to talk with and that will pray for you during this time. Appreciate and thank your friends for their concern and care.

Warning Signs

The typical warning signs that we hear about are the pain and or pressure in the chest, arms, and a cold sweat. Do you have, or have had any dizziness or weakness and or felt faint. These are things that I and others have ignored leading up to the scary ambulance drive to the emergency room.

I had had some pressure in my chest on several different occasions but had ignored it simply because I thought it would go away. Fortunately this thinking did not end my life but it could have. Ignoring any of these symptoms is very, very foolish.

Once the pressure had stayed with me overnight, only then I called my family doctor who of course instructed me to call 911 and not to come to their office. Please do not try to drive yourself to the hospital.

Our body is a wonderful system of miles of blood vessels that carry our life blood all over our body but for many reasons some of the main arteries can over time become clogged up and impede the flow of our blood. Our wonderful heart tries its best to compensate and keep the blood pumping perfectly but in the effort our blood pressure increases and over years this gets worse. My lack of quality care and my poor health lifestyle with years of elevated blood pressure contributed to my heart enlarging slightly which put more of a taxing load on my heart.

I had been to see my family doctor about high blood pressure. About a month previously, I had experienced shortness of breath and a nagging chest pressure as I went about my typical daily tasks. The pain was dull, more like a feeling of fullness or pressure. By the end of each day, it would usually disappear. I ignored the pain, hoping it would just go away. But one day, it remained with me through my working hours and into the evening. It was then that I decided to call my family doctor.

The call to 911 and the ride in the ambulance was to say the least not helping my problem.

At the emergency room the examination indicated that the results of an electrocardiogram, however, were not good. Previous electrocardiograms had been performed and the results then had been normal. The results now, however, were drastically different. "Robert, the tests indicate several obstructions of the coronary artery," my doctor said. "I want you to see a heart surgeon immediately, today."

So, three hours after my "routine" examination, I found myself undergoing a thorough cardiac examination and an exercise stress test. I did not take seeing a cardiologist lightly. But I did not believe there was anything seriously wrong, I was certain it was a mistake.

Like the electrocardiogram, the results of the stress test indicated a problem. I subsequently had coronary angiography that indicated three arterial blockages ranging from 50% to 95%. "You have CHD (coronary heart disease)," the cardiologist said. "I recommend coronary bypass surgery be done ASAP. At this moment you are a major heart attack just waiting to happen."

The shock of his words hit me like a slap in the face. This couldn't happen to me. I was not prepared to hear what he had to say; I had difficulty understanding. He was speaking about a heart problem—my heart problem! I could not accept this.

As I continued to listen numbly to the doctor, I was confused. Like most people, I knew something about the workings of the heart and the coronary arteries, but the information was minimal. It was not that information about the heart and heart disease was not available.

The American Heart Association, among others, had made available a tremendous amount of information. It had been of little interest to me. Such information, indeed the subject itself, was simply not relevant to my life. What did blocked arteries or heart attacks have to do with me?

In reality, what I didn't know could not only hurt me, it could kill me.

1. What I didn't know was that CHD usually develops silently, over a long period of time. Once it makes itself known, the primary result, a heart attack, is often immediately life threatening.

2. What I didn't know was that more than 10 million Americans have CHD and that every year; some 1.5 million people suffer a heart attack, causing 600,000 fatalities.

3. What I didn't know was that heart disease causes about 40% of all deaths in the United States each year, more than cancer, AIDS, auto accidents, and airplane disasters combined.

4. What I didn't know was that for about one third of heart attack victims, the first heart attack was the only one, resulting in sudden cardiac death.

5. What I didn't know was that while genetic history is important, most Americans with heart disease have it because of poor lifestyle habits involving diet, exercise, stress, and smoking.

Such information was simply outside the realm of my everyday life. But it all changed for me on that May afternoon. As the diagnosis sank in, ignorance ended for me. I was gripped by pure fear. At 58 years old, I had felt a kind of immortality that only the young experience. The concept of death had been a remote one. I pictured it at the end of a long life, after years of accomplishment, fulfillment, and joy. Old age was something that I looked forward to sharing with my wife. I had never contemplated the idea of death at a young age.

A decision was made to undergo coronary bypass surgery. I will go into more detail about the surgery later.

A few days after surgery, I went home to recover, happy to be alive and with my family again. But I was very concerned about my future. Surgery had circumvented the immediate problem of having a heart attack that ended my life. But my open heart surgery had not stopped the fact that my arteries could clog up again. Bypass did not "cure" me. My cardiologist told me. "You had heart disease the day before surgery, you had heart disease the day after surgery, and you have it today as well. The surgery took away the immediate threat but it did not remove the disease. Only a change in your lifestyle habits can possibly reduce your future heart attack risk."

So my doctor advised me:-

Don't smoke

Smoking is responsible for more than 500,000 deaths annually; smoking has historically been the single most preventable cause of death in the United States. Smoking contributes to about 30% of all cardiac deaths. Smokers are twice as likely as nonsmokers to have a heart attack and are five times more likely to die from sudden cardiac death.

Research shows that within 2 to 3 years of quitting, former smokers reduce their risk of heart attack and stroke to levels similar to those of people who never smoked. Within 5 years of quitting, former smokers have a 50% lower risk of heart attack than current smokers. The bottom line is that if you are not a smoker, don't start. If you are a smoker, get into a smoking cessation program.

Stress

There is considerable evidence that chronic stress may directly penalize cardiovascular health by raising cholesterol and blood pressure, promoting coronary inflammation, and triggering sudden cardiac death. While much more study needs to take place, there is a consensus about the indirect impact of daily stress: it can destroy healthy lifestyle habits.

When people are stressed it makes no difference how much they know about healthy living exercise is skipped, and cigarettes are smoked. If we have learned anything in the past 20 years of health it is this: understanding that smoking is unhealthy does not automatically lead to quitting smoking.

If stress cannot be reduced, it can be managed with techniques such as deep breathing, regular exercise, and meditation. Stress management is the key.

Exercise

The reality is that most Americans do not exercise. Fewer than 15% do it often enough or hard enough to produce cardiovascular benefits. Dr. Jeffrey Koplan, former director of the Centers for Disease Control and Prevention, said, "Physical inactivity, along with being overweight, accounts for more than 300,000 premature deaths each year in the United States."

This is a tragedy for heart health, as regular physical activity confers so many benefits. It strengthens the heart, boosts high-density lipoprotein cholesterol, reduces blood clotting, lowers blood pressure, aids in weight loss, maintains muscle strength, and helps to manage stress. A balanced exercise program should include daily physical activity (such as walking the dog), weight training for building strength, flexibility exercises (such as stretching or yoga) to prevent injury, and, most important, aerobic exercise to promote cardiovascular endurance and fat burning. Find a form of exercise that you like and will do. Brisk walking, jogging, aerobic dance, swimming, stair stepping, just do it regularly.

Do something every day. The key point is to encourage exercise.

Eat healthy food, but not too much of it

Perhaps nothing is more important for cardiac health than eating a healthy, balanced diet.

There are also problems with what we do not eat: some 40% of adults eat no fruit, 80% eat no whole grains, and 40% eat no vegetables.

The *Surgeon General's Report on Nutrition and Health* characterized Americans as "gobbling their way to the grave." It identified a causal link between the typical American diet and five of the 10 leading causes of death: CHD, cancer, high blood pressure, stroke, cirrhosis of the liver, and the nation's leading ailment, obesity.

There are many reasons behind such an unhealthy dietary pattern. Our fast-paced, out-of-time lifestyle has moved people away from shopping and cooking. Instead, they often eat on the run and settle for what is available, quickly, from restaurants, take-out places, and food stores. Many people have simply traded nutrition for convenience. "And when you add in what choices are available," according to Dr. Kelly Brownell, an obesity expert at Yale University, "the problem is compounded. We live in a toxic environment for making healthy food choices."

Moderate fat intake and when you eat fats, make them healthy ones such as olive oil; minimize unhealthy saturated and trans fats; center your diet on fruits, especially blueberries and pomegranates; whole grains, and vegetables; eat cardio protective foods such as oatmeal, fish, and nuts; eat lean meat; stay away from sugary desserts, soft drinks, and high-sodium foods; drink water; maybe an occasional glass of wine; choose low-fat dairy products; and choose whole foods over processed foods.

Second, eat real foods. We struggled in our house to eat healthy foods after my surgery, but these foods were often bland and tasteless. So we began to drift back to tastier, but unhealthier, foods.

Eating for heart health is not just about specific foods. It is also about how much is eaten. Unfortunately, we are eating a lot more than in the past. Restaurant meals and processed foods have become "super sized." Dinner plates now look like hubcaps. Most people have little understanding of portion size. A simple way to estimate healthy portions is to use your palm, fist, and thumb as a guide:

- 3 oz. The size of your palm is about the size of a 3-oz serving of cooked meat, fish, or poultry.
- 1 cup. One cup of cereal, spaghetti, potatoes, vegetables, or cut fruit is about the size of a woman's closed fist. A man's closed fist is about 1.5 cups.

- 1 teaspoon. One teaspoon of butter, peanut butter, mayonnaise, or sugar is about the size of the top joint of your thumb. Three such portions make up about 1 tablespoon.
- 1 handful = 1 oz. of snack food. For nuts or small candies, 1 handful equals about 1 oz. For chips or pretzels, 2 handfuls is about 1 oz.

Breakfast

In this fast-paced society, the day can get away from you. Under time pressure, the best-intended plans for healthy eating can go away. Eating a healthy breakfast, I can meet a good part of my nutritional needs even if the rest of the day gets messed up. I eat oatmeal topped with berries (strawberries, blueberries, or blackberries), chopped almonds or walnuts, and nonfat milk. It is a simple and easy way to get soluble fiber, antioxidants, vitamin D, omega-3 fatty acids, and calcium—a great nutritional start on the day. "Whatever you eat for the day, make certain you have a healthy breakfast."

Positive attitude

Creating a positive mindset is critical to long-term success. Patients who approach lifestyle change with hope and optimism do much better than those with a negative outlook.

A LAST WORD

Making healthy changes to benefit cardiovascular health is simple—not easy, but simple. Many patients can become discouraged, particularly if they have a lot to change or feel pressure to do it all at once. Advise them to make changes just for today. Don't fret about yesterday; it's over and you can't call it back. Don't be concerned with tomorrow, as it is not yet here. Instead, make a commitment to live healthy just for today. Pretty soon, the days will add up to weeks, months, and years, and changes will become habits. One day at a time.

Is Open-Heart Surgery Needed?

Open-heart surgery is any type of surgery where the chest is cut open and surgery is performed on the muscles, valves, or arteries of the heart.

According to the National Heart, Lung, and Blood Institute (NHLBI), coronary artery bypass grafting 5(CABG) is the most common type of heart surgery done on adults.

During this surgery, a healthy artery or vein is grafted (attached) to a blocked coronary artery. Typically veins (hopefully ones that are open and in good shape) will be taken from one of your legs and then this allows the grafted artery to "bypass" the blocked artery and bring fresh blood to the heart.

There are new heart procedures that can be performed with only small incisions. Consequently the term "open-heart surgery" can be misleading. However in my situation my chest was opened up.

Coronary heart disease occurs when the blood vessels that provide blood and oxygen for the heart muscle become narrow and hard. This is often called "hardening of the arteries."

Hardening occurs when fatty material forms a plaque on the walls of the coronary arteries. This plaque narrows the arteries, making it difficult for blood to get through. When blood can't flow properly to the heart, chest pains and or pressure often start and it can lead up to a heart attack.

Open-heart surgery can also be done to:
- repair or replace heart valves, which allow blood to travel through the heart
- repair damaged or abnormal areas of the heart
- implant medical devices that help the heart beat properly or if it stops beating (pace maker and a defibrillator)
- replace a damaged heart with a donated heart (heart transplantation)

The Procedure and Risks of Surgery

So how is open-heart surgery performed?

According to the National Institutes of Health, a CABG (coronary artery bypass grafting) takes from four to six hours. It is generally done following these basic steps:

- The patient is given general anesthesia. This ensures that the patient will be asleep and pain free through the whole surgery.
- The surgeon makes an 8- to 10-inch cut in the chest.
- The surgeon cuts through all or part of the patient's breastbone to expose the heart.
- Once the heart is visible, the patient may be connected to a heart-lung bypass machine. The machine moves blood away from the heart so that the surgeon can operate. Some of the newer procedures do not use this machine.
- The surgeon uses a healthy vein or artery, (typically from the leg, mine came from my right leg, below the knee on the left side) to make a new path around the blocked artery.
- The surgeon closes the breastbone with wire, leaving the wire inside the body.
- The original incision is stitched up.

Sometimes sternal plating is done for people at high-risk, such as people of advanced age or people who have had multiple surgeries. This is when the breastbone is rejoined with small titanium plates after the surgery.

What are the risks of open-heart surgery?

Risks for open-heart surgery include:
- chest wound infection (more common in patients with obesity or diabetes, or those who have had a CABG before)
- heart attack or stroke
- irregular heartbeat
- lung or kidney failure
- chest pain and low fever
- memory loss or "fuzziness"
- blood clots
- blood loss
- breathing difficulty

- pneumonia
- no improvement

According to the University of Chicago Medicine, the heart-lung bypass machine is associated with increased risks. These risks include stroke and memory problems.

Preparation

How do you prepare for open heart surgery?

Tell your doctor about any drugs you are taking, even over-the-counter medications, vitamins, and herbs. Inform them of any illnesses you have, including, herpes outbreak, cold, flu, or fever.

In the two weeks before the surgery, your doctor may ask you to quit smoking and stop taking blood-thinning medications, such as aspirin, ibuprofen, some supplements and or herbs. Tell your doctor everything you put in your mouth other than food.

It's important to talk to your doctor about your alcohol consumption before you prepare for the surgery. If you typically have three or more drinks a day and stop right before you go into surgery, you may go into alcohol withdrawal. This may cause life-threatening complications after open-heart surgery, including seizures or tremors. Your doctor can help you with alcohol withdrawal to reduce the likelihood of these complications.

The day before the surgery, you will be asked to wash yourself with a special anti-bacterial soap. This soap is used to kill bacteria on your skin and will lessen the chance of an infection after surgery. You will also be asked not to eat or drink anything after midnight prior to surgery. Your healthcare provider will give you more detailed instructions when you arrive at the hospital and are being prepped for surgery.

After Open-Heart Surgery

When you wake up after surgery, you will have two or three tubes in your chest. These are to help drain fluid from the area around your heart. You will have intravenous (IV) lines in your arm to supply you with fluids and medication, as well as a catheter (thin tube) in your bladder to remove urine.

You will also be attached to machines that monitor your heart. Nurses will be nearby to help you if something should arise.

You will usually spend at least your first night in the intensive care unit (ICU). You will then be moved to a regular care room for the next three to seven days.

I had a team of three nurses when I was in the ICU after surgery. According to my family they seemed to be exceptional.

Recovery, and What to Expect

How long does it take to fully recover from open heart surgery?

Expect a gradual recovery. It may take up to **six weeks** before you start feeling better, and up to **six months** to feel the full benefits of the surgery. However, the outlook is good for many people, and the grafts can work for many years. Nevertheless, surgery does not prevent artery blockage from happening again.

Taking care of yourself at home immediately after the surgery is an essential part of your recovery.

Incision care

Incision care is extremely important. Keep your incision site warm and dry, and wash your hands before and after touching it. If your incision is healing properly and there is no drainage, you can take a shower. The shower shouldn't be more than 10 minutes with warm (not hot) water. You should ensure that the incision site isn't hit directly by force of the water. It's also important to regularly inspect your incision sites for signs of infection, which include:

- increased drainage, oozing, or opening from the incision site
- redness around the incision
- warmth along the incision line
- fever

Pain management

Pain management is also incredibly important, as it can increase recovery speed and decrease the likelihood of complications like blood clots or pneumonia. You may feel muscle pain, throat pain, pain at incision sites, or pain from chest tubes. Your doctor will likely prescribe pain medication that you can take at home. It's important that you take it as prescribed. Some doctors may recommend taking the pain medication both before physical activity and before you sleep.

Get enough sleep

Some patients experience trouble sleeping after open-heart surgery, but it's important to get as much rest as possible. To get better sleep, you can:

- take your pain medication a half hour before bed
- arrange pillows to decrease muscle strain
- avoid caffeine, especially in the evenings

In the past, some have argued that open-heart surgery leads to a decline in mental functioning. However, most recent research has found that not to be the case. Though some patients may have open-heart surgery and experience mental decline later on, it's thought that this is most likely due to the natural effects of aging.

Some people may experience depression or anxiety after open-heart surgery. A therapist or psychologist can help you manage these effects. Be careful of getting attached to pain killers.

Rehabilitation

Open heart surgery and transplant patients are more susceptible to infection during their recovery.

Most people who've had a CABG benefit from participating in a structured, comprehensive rehabilitation program. This is usually done outpatient with visits several times a week. The program needs to include exercise, reducing risk factors, and dealing with stress, anxiety, and depression.

I found this to be very beneficial and the nurses were fantastic and helpful. They were special to me during my rehabilitation.

Can open heart surgery change your personality?

Although this condition, often referred to as "pump head," is usually short-lived, one study of bypass patients has suggested that the associated cognitive changes might worsen over time. Related research, however, indicates it is unlikely that cardiac surgery significantly alters how the brain works.

Some suggestions that I was given by the nurses at rehabilitation were:-

Step 1: Take one night at a time. Most bypass surgery patients experience sleep problems initially, according to surveys, with some finding that the problems become chronic.

Step 2: Face the pain head-on—both the physical and the emotional.

Step 3: Get out, even if only to the supermarket.

Step 4: Plan for doctor's appointments. Each doctor's visit can be filled with fear that you will fail your cardiac stress test or have a scan that would detect new blockages. I did not have confidence in my cardiologist at this time.

Step 5: Don't ignore the sex issues. Getting your doctor's OK to have sex after surgery is important.

Step 6: Learn to eat healthy.

Step 7: Arm yourself against toxic coworkers. Stepping back from a demanding job can be tough following heart surgery, but sometimes it's a necessity.

Again, expect a gradual recovery. It may take up to **six weeks** before you start feeling better, and up to **six months** to feel the full benefits of the surgery.

If you feel after six months that you have not improved get another doctor. Many times another perspective can make a big difference.

Remember taking care of yourself at home immediately after the surgery is an essential part of your recovery.

Activity and Driving

For the first 6 to 8 weeks, gradually build up your activity, such as doing household chores. In general, doctors recommend:
- Don't stand in one place longer than 20 minutes.
- Don't lift things that weigh more than 10 pounds.
- Don't push or pull heavy things.

Walk every day. Make three of those days a longer walk. Follow the guidelines the doctor or cardiac rehabilitation specialist gives you. Unless you've been told not to, you can climb stairs.

Your doctor will let you know when it's OK to drive again, usually within a month or so after surgery. It may be sooner if the surgeon did the operation with a just a small cut. There's no need to wait to ride as a passenger.

Diet

Get serious about eating healthy, but start gradually. For example start incorporating vegetables that are heart healthy in your diet. Beets, broccoli, cauliflower etc.
Add some specific fruit or fruit juice. One I will recommend is Pomagrate juice. I add a splash to some water or a little ginger ale. Did you know that pomegranate has many vitamins? Vitamin K has been said to be very good for your heart.

Healthy food choices help the healing process. Your doctor will let you know if you should have or avoid specific things.

You may not feel like eating for a while after your surgery. Try smaller meals, but more often.

If your appetite doesn't return within a few weeks, bring this up with your doctor.

Emotional Well-Being

It's common after heart surgery to be sad or blue, but these feelings should pass after the first few weeks. If they don't, talk to your doctor about it.

To keep your spirits up:
- Get dressed every day.
- Walk daily.
- Pick up your hobbies and social activities.
- Share your feelings with others.
- Get a good night's sleep.

Limit visits to 15 minutes at first. As you feel stronger and less tired, spend more time with your visitors.

Join a cardiac rehabilitation program or a support group.

Sources

SOURCES:
American Heart Association.
Answers by Heart. "How Can I Recover From Heart Surgery?"
American Heart Association, 2015.

Notes

The components of a rehabilitation program include exercise and the benefit from participating in a structured, comprehensive rehabilitation program, reducing risk factors, and dealing with stress, anxiety, and depression.

My participation was three times a week and it was a part of the hospital system where I had my open heart surgery. There were always three to five people trained in this program that were also qualified nurses. They were all exceptional and encouraging professionals.

I am convinced that my strength came back as I participated in this program.

As an un-expected bonus, my glucose reading came down and I was able to lower my medication. I later found that if I stopped my exercising the glucose became a problem again.

In the class room setting the education on eating healthy was very helpful and it has made me read the ingredients and the amount of saturated fat, sodium, and carbohydrates, and it was very shocking to see the marketing that the food companies use to keep us focused on the bad stuff.

My favorite was a Chicken Pot Pie that indicated on the package how many saturated fat grams, sugars and sodium were in the meal, though it was not clear that the amount that was high to start with was for only one half of the pie. Reading carefully we discovered that a serving size is only half of a pie.

I have to ask you how many will only eat half of the pie?

Another important tidbit post-surgery: have someone make sure your shower has been cleaned properly before you go back home and use it, and ask your doctor to recommend an anti-bacterial soap.

The class room time was very valuable but I disagree with the use of artificial sweeteners, but you must do your own research. The best option that I found was Stevia which does not raise my glucose. Secondly begin to detoxify yourself from all sugars. Much has been said about how addictive sugar really is. Some has said that it is likened to cocaine. When you try and quit the sugar habit you may agree. Gradually cut out the sugar. This is a great way to lose the weight and reduce the load on your heart.

Commitment to changing your lifestyle and getting exercise is crucial after heart surgery, and you must stay consistent. Remember the heart is a muscle. However let me caution you to sign up with a hospital sponsored program that has medical professionals monitoring all of what you do. They can monitor your heart rate, blood pressure and your glucose on the spot.

I was told that because of the number of blockages it would require that they do a quadruple by-pass.

It was a surprise to me for them not to try an alternative option as I did not have severe pains. Now I am in the hospital and all these tests have been done and I am told that a by-pass is my best course of action. It is here that you and I have to rely of the doctor's expertise.

In my case after a full six months I still had the pressure in my chest periodically and asked the cardiologist why this was still occurring. His reply was to say that they did their best and we will have to see what we can do with more and or different medications. This conversation went on for six more months with a few appointments along the way. I had the same conversation with this same doctor several times to no avail.

I then went to my family doctor and sternly requested he give me a referral to another heart doctor and after he realized that I was very serious I was able to see another heart doctor.

He was more concerned with improving my health and required some tests, such as an "echo cardiogram," and this showed that my heart was a little below thirty percent efficiency. He changed some of my medication and said he felt that I was a candidate for a "Defibrillator."

A couple months later I went into the hospital for a defibrillator/pacemaker. Since that time my heart has improved and it is a rare occasion that I have any discomfort from my heart, and it is related to over exerting.

The main point that I want to make here is that it is your life and health and if you are not happy and or feel that your care is not adequate then demand to see another qualified doctor.

Prepare your family members that the first time they see you if you are still the ICU you will looked like you are not doing well at all. But remember you have just had a major surgery.

My guess is that all the years I was treated by a family doctor with elevated blood pressure contributed to my enlarged heart. So it is important that if you keep visiting your doctor and your blood pressure stays high then demand to see a specialist.

At this point it is of course very, very helpful to have a family member or a close friend to remind you of what was said and your instructions. You will be given printed detail of what you can and cannot do.

Also if you are able to go to a rehabilitation program they will also remind you of things you should not be doing.

Conclusion

It is the author's (who is not a doctor or trained in health management) wish that this information will be some help as you prepare for heart surgery or during the recovery time after open heart surgery. Furthermore be encouraged that there has been so much advancement and improvement of open heart surgery in recent years. We have truly been blessed by all the wonderful doctors, nurses, technicians and scientists that have made great progress in this field.

Eat better, exercise, and do the research for a heart healthy diet.

Manage your stress and be encouraged that you are living in a time with so many modern procedures that will help you have a long productive life.

THE END

www.ingramcontent.com/pod-product-compliance
Lightning Source LLC
Chambersburg PA
CBHW081651220526
45468CB00009B/2618